March 25, 2023

Dear Grandchildren,

I hope you are all doing well. I am writing this letter (which appears to have turned into a booklet) today because most of you are now old enough to create children, and although this may not actually happen any time soon, I think you should be well informed for when the time does come. It's important to make the best health and wellness choices for your baby; this is important to me because your child will also be my great-grandchild. The younger two grandchildren will receive this letter when they are older. Hopefully the issues I'm addressing will have been resolved by then.

The following pages contain information I feel is important to bring to your attention. I know you don't need to know this information right now. You may choose to wait until your baby is on its way before you read it, or maybe you will choose not to have children; that's all fine. I think it's important for you to know about these issues because many parents aren't aware of these facts and consequently their children have health problems; many are serious. They think they are doing what is right but aren't aware of the scientific data and facts and unfortunately fall victim to unnecessary pain and suffering.

If you do choose to take a look at this information now, you may learn something that could help a friend or family member who currently do have a baby and/

or a young child.

When I was twenty-two I was married and had two children, your parents. I was clueless about children's healthcare, so we were always at the doctor's office. Back then it seemed everyone thought that the doctors and our healthcare systems knew what they were doing and would make sure we were taken care of properly. Looking back, I don't know if that was true, but I'm very happy your parents grew up without health complications.

A lot has changed since I was a child. When I was born, (in 1949) there were two vaccines available on the children's vaccine schedule. A child born today will receive seventy-three shots by the age of eighteen, according to the CDC children's vaccine schedule.

I didn't know about all this until I started looking into vaccines during the Covid 19 vaccine controversy. My eyes were opened by seeking a second opinion. I was shocked to find out what is currently happening in the vaccine industry, problems that could make a *big* difference in the future lives of children, your children, my great-grandchildren.

So what I am doing in this letter is giving you information in order for you to consider alternative ways to approach the possible vaccination of your children. The decision will be up to you, and I know you will do what you think is best.

I agree with the medical researcher Brucha Weisberger; "A parent who is willing to go against the popular narrative to research and discover what's safe and what isn't for their child, is someone deserving of the highest respect. The term "anti-vaxxer," while meant to be a slur, is actually the highest compliment." Don't let the government or pharmaceutical companies decide what is best for your child. Get all the information and decide for yourself. They don't love your child like you do, and they are willing to take risks with them that you may not want to take.

I've included graphs, links and references so you can find out more and verify this information; it's very important to be correctly informed and draw your own conclusions. This grandfather's conclusion is that all vaccines are harmful, many deadly. I'm interested to hear what you think.

I love you and care about you and your children. I want you and all our babies to live a happy and healthy life. Bringing a new life into this world is a special gift, we show our gratitude by being the best parent, grandparent or great-grandparent we can be.

As always, don't hesitate to ask questions.

Love,

G Father

P.S. I look forward to Emma and James III coming out to visit me this summer and I hope to see Ethan at Melina's graduation in May!

America's children are facing epidemics that the world has never seen. Chronic diseases are crippling our children in far greater numbers than in any generation in history, despite our "medical advancements." American children's ability to develop and thrive is being sabotaged by an avalanche of chronic ailments, with pediatric rates of some chronic conditions among the highest in the world.[1]

Behavioral and developmental disorders have become epidemic in our children. One in every six children today has been diagnosed with a developmental disability, such as autism, ADHD, or learning disabilities, according to research from the Centers for Disease Control and Prevention.

American children are the most highly vaccinated in the world. Currently, children receive repeated shots for 16 separate illnesses. Counting vaccines administered during pregnancy and yearly flu shots, by the time our children are 18 years old they will have received up to 73 doses of vaccines![2]

Robert F. Kennedy Jr. stresses in his article, *It's Time to Pay Real Attention to Children's Health*, that there is no crisis more urgent than the chronic illnesses now affecting over half of our nation's children.[3]

There are many issues with the vaccines. The three I will address with you at this time are: *safety*, *aluminum* in vaccines, and better health outcomes with *no vaccines*.

How safe are the vaccines?

Deciding to inject a product into yourself or your child's body is an important decision. Here are some facts you should know before making that decision.

1. *Immunity from Liability for Vaccine Harms.* By the early 1980s, pharmaceutical companies faced crippling liability for injuries to children caused by their vaccines.[4] Instead of letting these market forces drive them to develop safer vaccines, Congress passed the National Childhood Vaccine Injury Act (the 1986 Act) which eliminated pharmaceutical company liability for injuries caused by their vaccine products.[5]

2. *Pharmaceutical Company Misconduct.* Before 1986, Merck, GSK, Sanofi and Pfizer paid billions of dollars for misconduct and injuries related to their drug products.[6] These same companies sell almost all childhood vaccines, but because of the 1986 Act, they now cannot be held accountable for misconduct and injuries from their vaccine products.

3. *Pediatric Vaccine Clinical Trials Lack Placebos and Are Too Short.* The pivotal clinical trials relied upon to license childhood vaccines do not include a placebo-control group and safety review periods which are the standard for scientific testing. They are also typically only days or months long.[7] The safety profile for a pediatric vaccine is therefore not known before it is licensed and routinely used in children.[8] You're basically giving your child untested injections, but because they are on the children's vaccine schedule, the vaccine companies automatically make billions of dollars and are not responsible for any problems the vaccines may cause.

4. *Autism.* Autism is the most controversial of the claimed vaccine injuries for children and the one HHS and CDC declare they have thoroughly studied. Most parents with autistic children claim vaccines -- including DTaP, Hep B, Hib, PCV13, and IPV, each injected 3 times by 6 months -- are the cause of their child's autism.[9] The CDC tells these parents that "Vaccines Do Not Cause Autism."[10]

The CDC was recently sued for copies of the studies which they claim support that these vaccines do not cause autism.[11] In the end, the CDC identified 20 studies, 18 of which studied a different vaccine (MMR[12]) or an ingredient not in these vaccines (thimerosal), and one irrelevant study regarding antigens.[13] Incredibly, the final study the CDC identified explained that it searched for but failed to identify any study to support that DTaP does *not* cause autism.[14] The same is true for Hep B, Hib, PCV13, and IPV.[15] Worse, HHS's primary autism expert in Vaccine Court testified that vaccines can cause autism in some children.[16] Given the lack of studies regarding vaccines and autism, it should not be surprising that few or no studies support the CDC's other vaccine safety claims.

According to The Autism Society, "Autism spectrum disorder (ASD) is a complex developmental disability; signs typically appear during early childhood and affect a person's ability to communicate and interact with others. ASD is defined by a certain set of behaviors and is a 'spectrum condition' that affects individuals differently and to varying degrees." Some of the behaviors associated with autism include:

- Delayed speech or absence of speech
- Difficulty making eye contact or holding a conversation
- Difficulty with executive functioning
- Narrow, intense interests
- Poor motor skills
- Sensory sensitivities
- Repetitive behaviors

It's important to note that individuals with autism may exhibit all or some of these behaviors, in addition to many others.

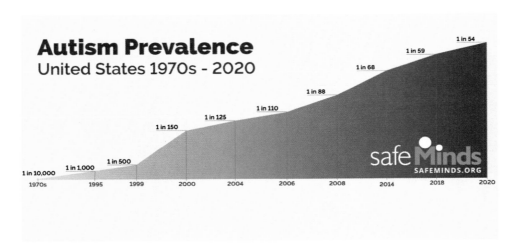

As you can see by this chart that summarizes the data, 1 in every 54 children had autism in 2020, the 2021 report shows 1 in every 44, and in the 1960's autism didn't even exist. If autism continues to accelerate at its current rate, by 2025, 1 in every 4 children in the United States will have autism.

Aluminum in vaccines.

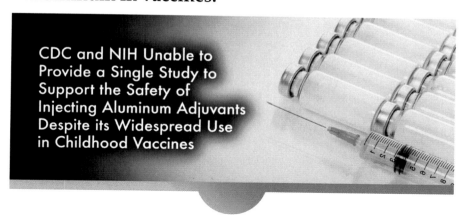

CDC and NIH Unable to Provide a Single Study to Support the Safety of Injecting Aluminum Adjuvants Despite its Widespread Use in Childhood Vaccines

CDC and NIH's responses to ICAN's Freedom of Information Act (FOIA) requests regarding aluminum adjuvant reveal a stunning admission: they do not have a single study to support the safety of recommending repeated injection of this cyto- and-neuro toxic substance as part of the CDC's childhood vaccine schedule.

To view the full report and law suit visit: https://icandecide.org/press-release/cdc-and-nih-unable-to-provide-a-single-study-to-support-the-safety-of-injecting-aluminum-adjuvants-despite-its-widespread-use-in-childhood-vaccines/

Recently new technology has revealed to scientists previously unknown information about the amount of aluminum in the human body and how it affects our health. Since this new data exposes that there is a serious problem with aluminum exposure, the people that sell us aluminum products are trying to hide this information.

The following article explains the facts about what the scientific research reveals and the many possible consequences of injecting aluminum into the body, especially for children.

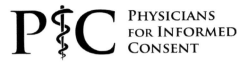

PHYSICIANS FOR INFORMED CONSENT

Delivering Data on Infectious Diseases & Vaccines™

ALUMINUM IN VACCINES
What Parents Need to Know

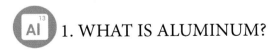 ## 1. WHAT IS ALUMINUM?

Aluminum is a silvery-white, moldable, and durable light metal. These qualities make it useful in numerous industries and products, including machinery, construction, storage, cookware, eating utensils, textiles, dyes, and cosmetics. Aluminum is also the most abundant metal in the earth's crust, and virtually all aluminum in the environment is in the soil. However, aluminum is not naturally found in significant amounts in living organisms (such as plants and animals), and aluminum has no known biological function. During the past century, aluminum usage in certain products has led to higher human exposure. The greatest sources of such exposure are aluminum-containing foods (e.g., baking powder, processed foods, infant formulas, etc.), cookware, medical products (e.g., antiperspirants, antacids, etc.), allergy shots, and vaccines.[1-3]

 ## 2. WHY IS ALUMINUM IN VACCINES?

Certain vaccines use aluminum compounds (i.e., aluminum hydroxide and aluminum phosphate) as adjuvants, ingredients that enhance the immune response to an antigen (foreign substance).[4,5] The U.S. Food and Drug Administration (FDA) states that if some vaccines did not include aluminum, the immune response they trigger may be diminished.[6]

3. WHICH VACCINES CONTAIN ALUMINUM?

The following vaccines contain aluminum and are administered to infants, children and adolescents (Fig. 1):

• Hepatitis B (HepB)

• Diphtheria, tetanus, and pertussis (whooping cough) (DTaP and Tdap)

• Haemophilus influenzae type b (PedvaxHIB)

• Pneumococcal (PCV)

• Hepatitis A (HepA)

• Human papillomavirus (HPV)

• Meningococcal B (MenB)

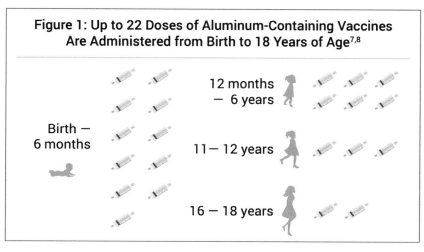

Figure 1: Up to 22 Doses of Aluminum-Containing Vaccines Are Administered from Birth to 18 Years of Age[7,8]

 4. IS EXPOSURE TO ALUMINUM SAFE?

The FDA has considered aluminum to be generally recognized as safe (GRAS) since 1975.[9] However, before 1990, the technology did not exist to accurately detect small quantities of aluminum administered to subjects in scientific studies.[10] Consequently, the amount of aluminum that could be absorbed before the onset of negative effects was not known.

Since 1990, due to advancements in technology, small amounts of aluminum that remain in the human body have been observed to interfere with a variety of cellular and metabolic processes in the nervous system and in tissues of other parts of the body.[1,10,11] The greatest negative effects of aluminum have been observed in the nervous system and range from motor skill impairment to encephalopathy (altered mental state, personality changes, difficulty thinking, loss of memory, seizures, coma, and more).[2,12]

The U.S. Department of Health and Human Services (HHS) recognizes aluminum as a known neurotoxin.[2] (substance that alters the structure or function of the nervous system) In addition, the FDA has warned about the risks of aluminum toxicity in infants and children.[13]

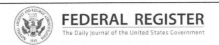

FEDERAL REGISTER
The Daily Journal of the United States Government

"Term infants with normal renal function may also be at risk because of their rapidly growing and immature brain and skeleton, and an immature blood-brain barrier. Until they are 1 to 2 years old, infants have lower glomerular filtration rates than adults, which affects their kidney function. The agency is concerned that young children and children with immature renal function are at a higher risk resulting from any exposure to aluminum."

— U.S. Food and Drug Administration (FDA), June 2003[13]

5. HOW MUCH ORAL ALUMINUM IS UNSAFE?

In 2008, the Agency for Toxic Substances and Disease Registry (ATSDR), a division of HHS, used studies of the neurotoxic effects of aluminum to determine that no more than 1 milligram (mg) (1,000 micrograms [mcg]) of aluminum per kilogram (kg) of body weight should be taken **orally** per day to avoid aluminum's negative effects.[2]

 6. HOW MUCH INJECTED ALUMINUM IS UNSAFE?

To determine the amount of aluminum that can be safely injected requires a conversion of the ATSDR oral aluminum limit. The ATSDR oral aluminum limit is based on 0.1% of oral aluminum being absorbed into the bloodstream, as the digestive tract blocks nearly all oral aluminum (Fig. 2a).[2] In contrast, aluminum injected intramuscularly bypasses the digestive tract, and 100% of aluminum may be absorbed into the bloodstream over time (i.e., the proportion of absorbed aluminum is 1,000 times greater). To account for these different absorption amounts, the ATSDR oral aluminum limit must be divided by 1,000.

This conversion results in an ATSDR- derived bloodstream aluminum limit of 1 mcg of aluminum (0.1% of 1,000 mcg) per kg of body weight per day (Fig. 2b). Consequently, to avoid the neurotoxic effects of aluminum, no more than 1 mcg of aluminum per kg of body weight should enter the bloodstream on a daily basis. Figure 3 shows the ATSDR-derived bloodstream aluminum limit for infants of various ages based on their weight.

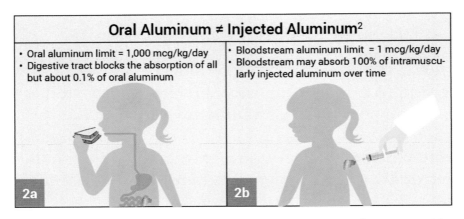

Oral Aluminum ≠ Injected Aluminum²

• Oral aluminum limit = 1,000 mcg/kg/day • Digestive tract blocks the absorption of all but about 0.1% of oral aluminum	• Bloodstream aluminum limit = 1 mcg/kg/day • Bloodstream may absorb 100% of intramuscularly injected aluminum over time

2a · 2b

Figures 2a, 2b: When taken orally, only about 0.1% of aluminum is able to enter the bloodstream through the digestive tract (2a). In contrast, when intramuscularly injected, the proportion of aluminum that enters the bloodstream over time is 1,000 times greater (100%) because the digestive tract is bypassed (2b).

 ## 7. HOW MUCH ALUMINUM IS IN VACCINES?

The amount of aluminum in vaccines varies.[16] In 1968, the federal government set the limit for the amount of aluminum in vaccines to 850 mcg per dose based on the amount of aluminum needed to make certain vaccines effective.[6,17] Consequently, the amount of aluminum in aluminum-containing childhood vaccines ranges from 125 to 850 mcg per dose. Figure 4 shows the aluminum content of one dose of various vaccines administered to children.

3 · ATSDR-Derived Bloodstream Aluminum Limit[2,14,15]

	Newborn	3.3 micrograms/day
	2 months	5.3 micrograms/day
	4 months	6.7 micrograms/day
	6 months	7.6 micrograms/day
	12 months	9.3 micrograms/day

Figure 3: This chart shows the aluminum limit for infants of various ages, as derived from the Agency for Toxic Substances and Disease Registry, a division of the U.S. Department of Health and Human Services. The limit indicates that *no more than 1 mcg of aluminum per kg of body weight should enter the bloodstream* on a daily basis to avoid the neurotoxic effects of aluminum.

 8. HAVE ANY STUDIES COMPARED THE AMOUNT OF ALUMINUM IN VACCINES TO THE ATSDR-DERIVED LIMIT?

A recent study that intended to compare the amount of aluminum in vaccines to the ATSDR-derived bloodstream limit was published in 2011.[18] However, this study incorrectly based its calculations on 0.78% of oral aluminum being absorbed into the bloodstream rather than the value of 0.1% used by the ATSDR in its computations.[19,20] As a result, the 2011 study assumed that nearly 8 (0.78%/0.1%) times more aluminum can safely enter the bloodstream, and this led to an incorrect conclusion.

9. IS EXPOSURE TO ALUMINUM FROM VACCINES SAFE?

Vaccines are injected intramuscularly, and the rate at which aluminum from vaccines migrates from human muscle to the bloodstream is not known. Studies in animals suggest that it can take from a couple of months to more than a year for aluminum from vaccines to enter into the bloodstream, due to multiple variables.[21-23] Because *the cumulative aluminum exposure from vaccines in children less than 1 year old exceeds the ATSDR-derived daily limit by several hundreds* (Figs. 3 and 4), the limit would still be exceeded if aluminum from vaccines entered the bloodstream over the course of about a year. Moreover, studies have shown that aluminum from vaccines is absorbed by immune cells that travel to distant parts of the body, including the brain.[24]

Studies have also shown that adverse effects of aluminum in vaccines may not be restricted to neurological conditions. A study published in Academic Pediatrics found that asthma occurred in 1 in 183 vaccinated children for every 1 mg (1,000 mcg) increase in aluminum exposure.[25]

The extent of the negative effects of aluminum in vaccines is not known, as safety studies comparing a population vaccinated with aluminum-containing vaccines to a population not vaccinated with such vaccines have not been conducted.

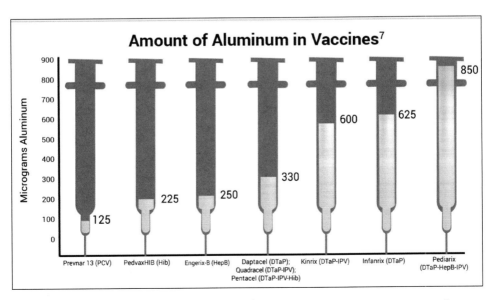

Figure 4: This graph shows the aluminum content of one dose of various vaccines administered to children. The

administration of one dose each of Prevnar 13, PedvaxHIB, Engerix-B, and Infanrix at one visit delivers 1,225 mcg of aluminum. PCV, Hib, HepB, and DTaP vaccines are administered multiple times by 6 months of age. The rate at which aluminum from vaccines migrates from human muscle to the bloodstream is not known.

All references are available at: physiciansforinformedconsent.org/aluminum.

Better health outcomes with no vaccines?

This is the third and final issue I will be explaining in this letter. Although the previous issues are very concerning, this one really lets you know what's actually happening to children in the United States today.

Please pay close attention to this information and if you have any doubts about its authenticity, just follow the references and get the data from these scientifically proven outcomes.

Pierre Kory, MD MPA ✔ @PierreK... · 3h ···
I stand by this statement and will do so to my grave. If I had young children today, not one would get even a single childhood vaccine. Thank you Twitter for allowing me to publicly state my data-driven & highly researched interpretation of vaccine (non) science. 🧵

ılıl 48.6K 💬 95 ↻ 353 ♡ 1,816 ⬆

Dr. Kory is the former Chief of the Critical Care Service and Medical Director of the Trauma and Life Support Center at the University of Wisconsin. He is a Board-Certified Specialist in Critical Care Medicine, Pulmonary Diseases, and Internal Medicine. He is most known for his specialty as one of the international pioneers in the development and teaching of Critical Care Ultrasonography. He is the senior editor of the most popular and award-winning textbook in that field, and the 2nd edition of his book has now been published in 7 languages.

Dr. Kory is only one of many highly qualified doctors (some are the most highly qualified doctors in their field of expertise) exposing what they have discovered about the childhood vaccine schedule created by the CDC.

"Pre-Covid, me and my beautiful family were fully vaxxed. Covid led me to research vaccine science. This effort transformed my perception of vaccines & revealed decades of corruption in the medical sciences and the vaccination industry.

Pro-vaccine propaganda has been immensely successful for many decades and ended up literally defining the field of Pediatrics. The idea that vaccines are the backbone of historic improvements in population health is built on myths. Immense data supports my conclusion."   Dr. Kory

There are many qualified scientific papers, books and articles showing the same results (most from other countries). One good example is a pediatrician in Oregon, Dr. Paul Thomas.

Dr. Thomas had noticed that the unvaccinated children rarely came in for office visits compared to the vaccinated children. He wrote a book about what he had discovered called "The Vaccine-Friendly Plan." The Oregon Medical Board didn't like that Dr. Thomas was suggesting an alternative to the CDC children's vaccine schedule and told him to prove he was correct. So Dr. Paul Thomas had a professional scientific study done on the data he had collected from patients in his practice.

The purpose was to see how the health of the children whose parents had chosen to vaccinate them compared with those who weren't vaccinated. The results were amazing, even to Dr. Thomas, but instead of thanking Dr. Thomas for bringing this to their attention, the Oregon Medical Board yanked his medical license.

You can view a video in which Dr. Thomas explains his own findings, and then presents other studies which reached the same conclusions. You can use the following link or QR code.

https://rumble.com/v106qn9-stunning-dr.-paul-thomas-blows-up-the-conventional-vaccine-narrativeincredi.html

The next pages contain a summary of Dr. Thomas's data demonstrated by his graphs. These graphs were created from the data collected in Dr. Thomas's pediatric practice from a child's birth to 9.5 years of age. Fortunately these graphs are easy to understand and clearly demonstrate the current status of the health condition of children in the United States.

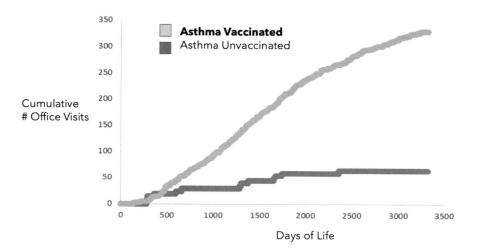

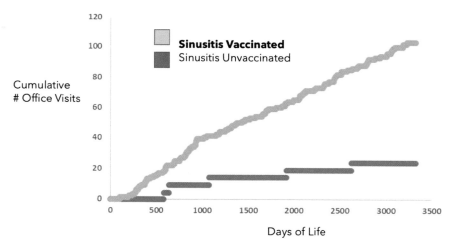

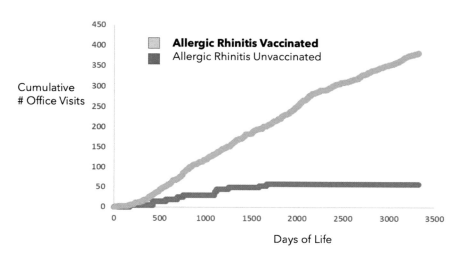

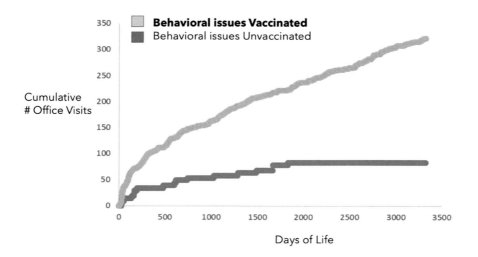

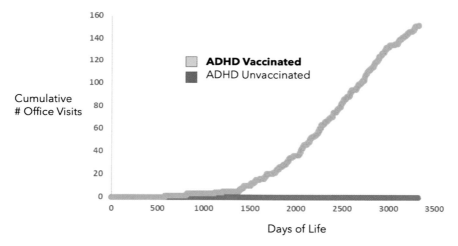

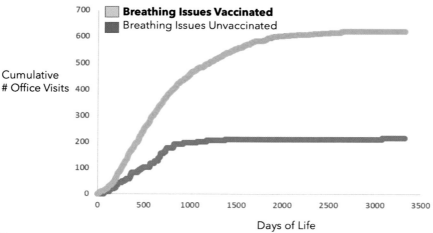

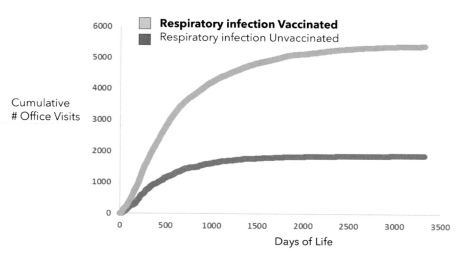

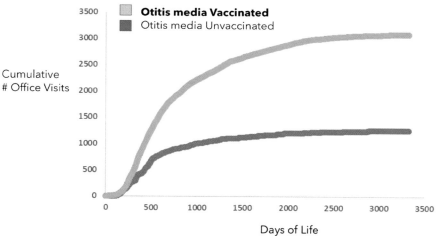

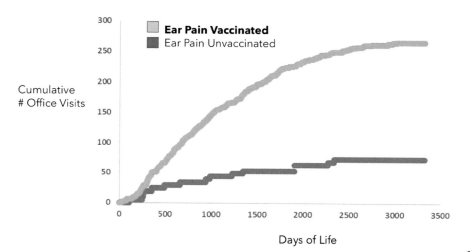

19

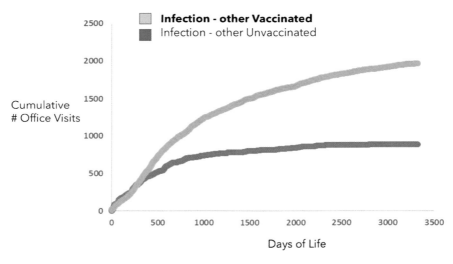

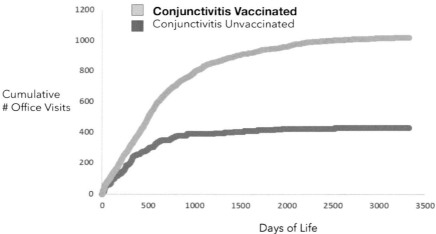

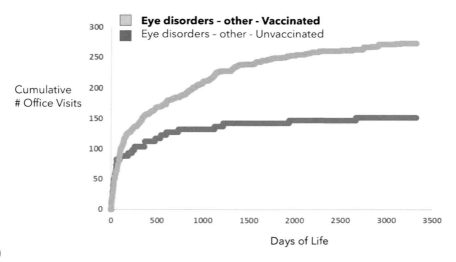

20

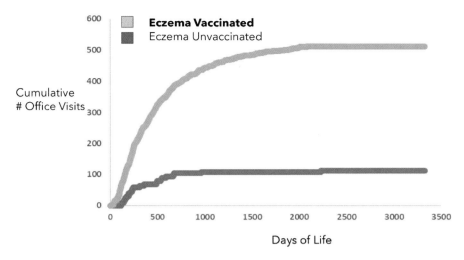

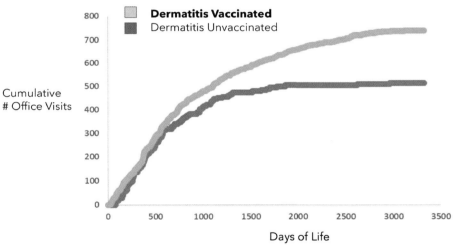

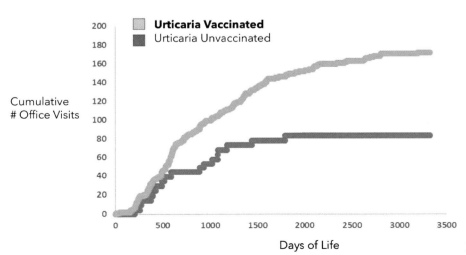

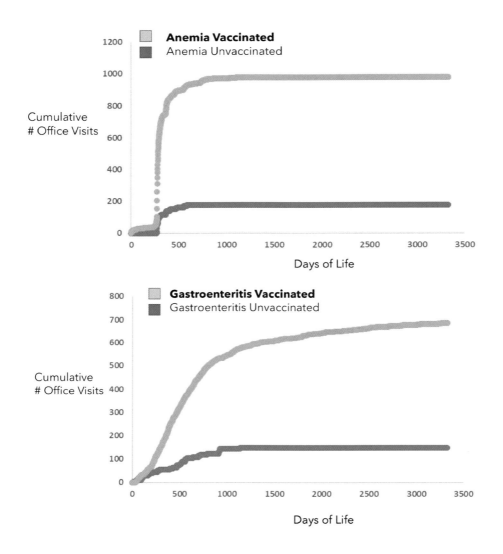

You might want to read the financial incentives paper that showed Dr Paul's clinic was losing over $1 million a year in just lost administration fees from those parents who chose not to do some or all the vaccines. Per Dr. Thomas, "It is very profitable for a pediatric practice to follow and push the CDC schedule. In fact I bet most, if not all, practices would not survive without that income. Is it any wonder why practices now discharge patients who won't follow the CDC schedule?"

Conclusion

There have been many books and scientific papers written to show the problems with the CDC childhood schedule. I have just offered you a sample to let you know there is much to consider before you let someone inject foreign objects into your new baby's pure body.

The first day of life, a Hep B vaccine is given to a newborn. Hepatitis B is a vaccine-preventable liver infection caused by the hepatitis B virus (HBV). Hepatitis B is spread when blood, semen, or other body fluids from a person infected with the virus enters the body of someone who is not infected. This can happen through sexual contact, sharing needles, syringes, or other drug-injection equipment, or from mother to baby at birth. Hep B testing is done to every mother before giving birth, so why do all babies receive this vaccine? United States now has the highest "day of birth" death rate, higher than all the other developed countries combined.

Some say that the pharmaceutical companies have developed the childhood vaccines to create these problems so they can later sell the vaccinated their drugs to cover up some of the symptoms and seemingly help but not cure the problem; this creates a lifelong profit flow. This has not been proven, but it's obvious that something like this could be true.

I could go on and on, but I hope you get the idea. My concern is to help prevent unnecessary harm to your children because you didn't know about these issues. I hope this information will inspire you to find out if your child really needs these dangerous vaccines. Unfortunately our society has let this happen, but now that you know about our current lack of safety protocols and the pharmaceutical industry's corruption, you can save your children from this unnecessary harm, and possibly save their life, if you choose.

REFERENCES

[1] https://www.ncbi.nlm.nih.gov/books/NBK92197/

[2] https://www.healthychildren.org/English/Pages/default.aspx

[3] https://childrenshealthdefense.org/news/time-pay-real-attention-childrens-health/

[4] https://www.nap.edu/read/2138/chapter/2#2("The litigation costs associated with claims of damage from vaccines had forced several companies [by 1986] to ... stop producing already licensed vaccines.")

[5] 42 U.S.C. § 300aa-11 "No person may bring a civil action ... in the amount greater than $1,000 ... against a vaccine administrator or manufacturer ... for damages arising from a vaccine-related injury or death."); Bruesewitz v. Wyeth LLC, 562 U.S. 223, 243 (2011) ("the [1986] Act preempts all design-defect claims against vaccine manufacturers brought by plaintiffs who seek compensation for injury or death caused by vaccine side effects")

[6] https://www.citizen.org/sites/default/files/2408.pdf

[7-8] https://icandecide.org/hhs/ICAN-Reply.pdf (see Section I)

[9] https://www.ncbi.nlm.nih.gov/pubmed/16685182; https://www.ncbi.nlm.nih.gov/pubmed/25398603; https://www.ncbi.nlm.nih.gov/pubmed/16547798; https://www.ncbi.nlm.nih.gov/pmc/articles/PMC1448378/

[10] https://www.cdc.gov/vaccinesafety/concerns/autism.html

[11] https://bit.ly/3d0brl4

[12] https://www.c-span.org/video/?c4546421/rep-bill-posey-calling-investigation-cdcs-mmr-reasearch-fraud

[13] https://www.icandecide.org/wp-content/uploads/2020/03/Stipulation-and-Order-Fully-Executed.pdf

[14] https://www.nap.edu/read/13164 chapter/12?term=autism#545

[15] https://icandecide.org/hhs/ICAN-Reply.pdf (see Section VI)

[16] http://icandecide.org/documents/zimmerman.pdf

Made in the USA
Las Vegas, NV
28 June 2023

74022542R00019